A practical guide with inspirational real life stories that will make you laugh and cry.

This remarkable collection captures the grand achievements and every-day victories of our resilient peers.

Profits from the sale of this book will be donated to various organizations dedicated to helping those living with Parkinson.

To order: www.createspace.com/3747802

All rights reserved. No parts of this book may be reproduced, stored in a retrieval system or transmitted in any form or by any means without the prior written permission of the publishers, except by a reviewer who may quote brief passages in a review to be printed in a newspaper, magazine or journal.
Disclaimer: This book is not intended to dispense medical advice. Consult your physician prior to making any changes to your treatment.
Chris Ludwig, @2011

Passages Press
Osprey, FL 34229

Dear Reader

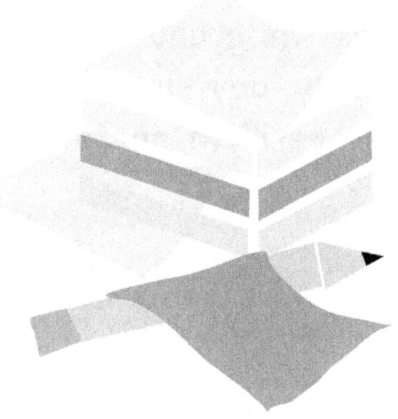

Dear Reader –

We had uncertain expectations when we first decided to record our Parkinson experiences in a journal. Our hope was that it would be filled with precocious wisdom and sage advice, and occasionally we surprised even ourselves with our heartwarming recollections. We also realized that some of the most effective pieces contained practical advice that, while not genius – was certainly helpful!

This first volume contains examples of the joy, the frustration, the confusion and determination, the innermost thoughts, of people who have been diagnosed with Parkinson Disease. You will find advice from the heart to others who share our plight, and private remembrances of the small victories and defeats you're sure to encounter.

This book is the result of a collaborative effort of relative strangers whose viewpoints and experiences were so different; and yet, they found common ground in the strength and courage they all exhibited. You will be moved in different ways by their stories. Writing them became therapeutic; reading them became inspirational. We hope that you find wisdom, spirit, and positive "vibes", as well as inspiration that guides you through your personal journey.

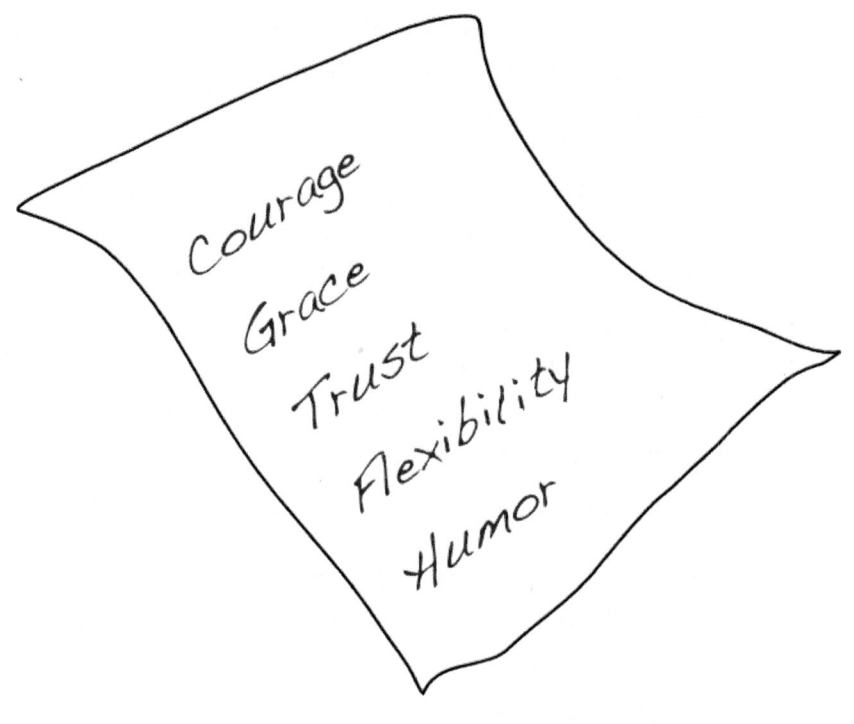

Table of Contents

Dear Reader……………………………………………….2

    Who Are We?..10

    Our Meeting……………………………………….14

Questionnaire……………………………………………20

    Thoughts on Adjusting to Your New Reality……….34

Early PD (Up to 10 Years)……………………………....44

    The Diagnosis 1,2,3……………………………….46

    Accepting the Diagnosis (or not) & Coping……….. 68

Mid PD (10 + Years)………………………………….. 72

    Care Givers, Doing Angles Work………………….76

    We Have Lots of Company………………………..80

    Exercise is Medicine…………………………….....92

Later PD (15+ Years)………………………………......96

    Goodbye Wheels…………………………………..100

    Striking the Right Balance………………………...104

    Impromptu Gym Drill Workout……………….....109

What Now? – Dave and Chris – In Summary….......117

Parkinson Basics

There are a few things you may wish to keep in mind about the Parkinson "Movers and Shakers" book. It is the result of collaboration and reflects a deep commitment to help others through the ordeal of living with Parkinson Disease (PD). The authors realized that although they were not equally knowledgeable about all facets of the disease, they all had access to many resources, thanks to the Neuro Challenge Foundation, including the results of a detailed questionnaire that was completed by fellow PDers. Thanks to those who assisted in the gathering of information for our edification. Here's some basic operating information:

Parkinson Disease is a progressive neurological disorder for which there is no known cure (yet). Other neurological disorders include MS (Multiple Sclerosis) and ALS (Lou Gehrig's disease). PD symptoms result from a lack of dopamine in the system; they include tremors, stiffness, ranging from awkward movements to the limbs freezing in place for periods of time. As the disease progresses, other internal organs may become involved. Medication currently helps to mask the symptoms; as the disease progresses dosages may have to be increased. Treatment for the early phases of PD consists of largely juggling several different medications; the effectiveness and variety of these new medications provide far better relief with fewer side effects.

One major difference among PD patients is the pace at which the disease progresses. It is different for each individual. Look at Michael J Fox, Mohammed Ali, Yasser Arafat, and Pope John Paul II. In most cases, the disease progresses slowly, but, not in all.

Every effort was made to be sure the outlook that was reflected was realistic, and presented a fair picture. While medications have been developed to slow PD down, there is no cure. (Yet!) A lot of the research into PD has been focused on treating the symptoms and to slow PD down. But there continues to be major efforts underway to find a cure.

First steps in our communications effort included the development and distribution of a questionnaire soliciting real life information from numerous current Parkinson patients and their caregivers, which provided a broad perspective, as well as a detailed focus on the differences and similarities of Parkinson progress. The responses were thoughtful and frank. With PD there is a spectrum of symptoms that occur unpredictably, and affect each individual differently; there are also strong similarities in support needs. We all want quick access to practical information that will help us cope, and we want to learn about ways to embrace hope and to "accentuate the positive".

So, you'll find helpful insights about how others cope with the symptoms and side-effects, tried and true helpful hints, customized exercises, and true moving personal stories that will inspire you.

As you read, you will find Journal Entry pages. Since we learned that several readers took notes, we provided a place to keep them. Surprisingly, each person used them differently; some kept cryptic notes to supplement their retention, others wrote philosophical notes to come back to again, and still others found them as a valuable place to keep follow-on details. One reader said she reread them every few months to see how her viewpoint and support needs changed over time. We hope you will find them helpful.

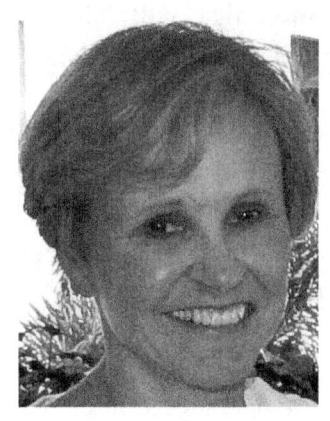

Who Are We?

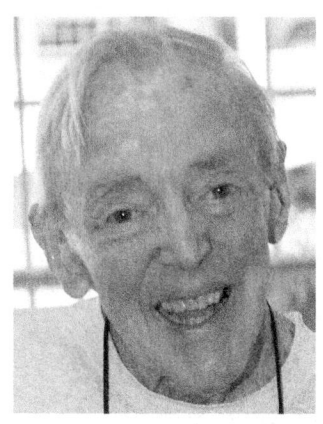

Chris Ludwig was Vice President of technology for a major financial institution in the Northeast. Her job entailed international travel, including an unforgettable year spent in Ireland. While travelling, she noticed a tremor in her right hand and was told it probably was an "Essential Tremor", a condition considered by some to be a "health nuisance". Since it can also be an early symptom of Parkinson, her doctor told her to check it out with a specialist. She chose to believe the essential tremor diagnosis, until her personal physician insisted that she see a Neurologist for confirmation. She was greatly disappointed when the doctor diagnosed her with Parkinson's as well as Essential Tremor.

Chris is an avid exercise practitioner, and believes strongly that "Exercise is medicine!" She chose to have Deep Brain Stimulation surgery, but had to discontinue the treatment because of some healing issues. She and her doctor are presently deciding "What's next?"

Chris now lives and shakes in Florida and Cape Cod with her husband Dale, where she continues to appreciate every day with joy and enthusiasm.

Dave Anderson was born and raised a small town boy, and ultimately worked in a challenging environment in international advertising with a Fortune 500 company. After taking early retirement he noticed a slight tremor in his left hand, which was diagnosed as PD. His personal journey through the disbelief, anger and denial affected his outlook and that of his support group. Working together with a personal trainer, Wayne McKenna, a rigorous training program was put in place, which Dave credits with not only slowing the progress of PD, but actually reducing some of his symptoms. Dave's passionate commitment was "ahead of his time"; studies done since then indicate that there are many benefits to patients who are faithful to physical fitness. The program and Dave's developing friendship with Wayne had a profoundly positive effect on Dave's attitude and consequently his symptoms. The results, both physical and psychological led Dave to write "How to Tame Parkinson's by Keeping Fit," released in 2005, which chronicles Dave's criteria for selecting a personal trainer and developing exercise routines for the various stages of Parkinson Disease.

His ability to capture his feelings has provided us with an appreciation for the difficulties of having an unpredictable disease; he also was able to lift our spirits at the wonder and inner strength he exhibits. And when Dave and Wayne met Vince Doherty they appreciated his fresh viewpoint and perspective. He participated in many planning meetings and brought a different view to the discussions about content

There were so many people who helped us in every facet of this project, from information gathering to support, to providing us with access to their professional networks, to just plain cheerleading. We were overwhelmed by how often the first kind response to a request was, "I know someone who was just diagnosed – how can I help?" We found the same unselfish attitude and spirit in the larger Parkinson community. Thanks to each and every one of you.

"I know someone who was just diagnosed – how can I help?"

Our Meeting

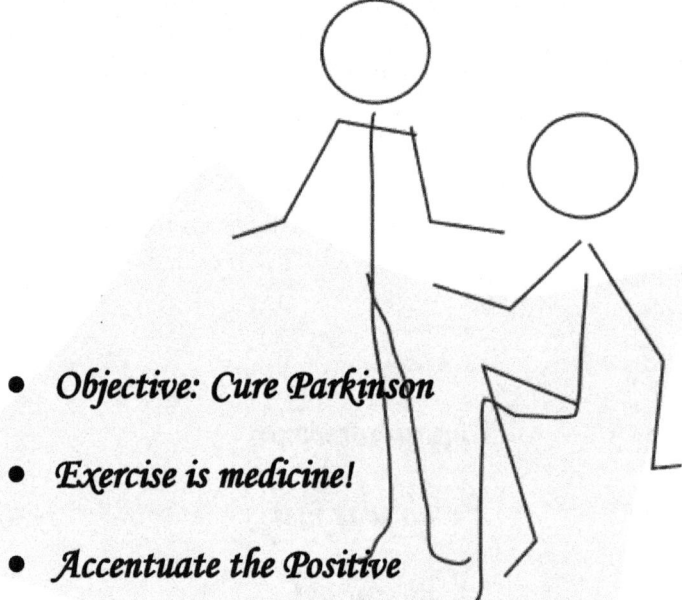

- *Objective: Cure Parkinson*
- *Exercise is medicine!*
- *Accentuate the Positive*

Up until 3 years ago, Dave Anderson, Vince Doherty, and Chris Ludwig were strangers. What they all had in common was a Parkinson diagnosis. Now when they meet to work on their book project, they find trust and support ... and real admiration for each other's achievements, no matter how big or small. They all believe that this was meant to be – and that they are fortunate to be part of this effort. Ironically, it was a search for a book that made their paths cross. Dave, and Wayne his Personal Trainer, worked together and published a book about exercise and Parkinson Disease. Check it out at www.tamingparkinsons.com.

They didn't know they were searching – but here's how they each found the others. First, Vince's story-

"As a Christmas present, my wife gave me a membership in the Sarasota YMCA, where she noticed a book on sale, which highlighted an exercise program developed by Dave Anderson and his personal trainer, named Wayne McKenna.

I looked up Mr. McKenna and arranged for him to put a program together for me. Learning the program and seeing the faith and work ethic of Dave has given me the strength to continue on. I am convinced that with regular exercise, concentrated on the body's "core", and on balance, Parkinson's progress will be slowed."

Dave and Wayne have become Parkinson "exercise experts" and have published their exercise routines. Both believe that strenuous and regular workouts have slowed the progress of PD.

Dave first met Vince while working out.

"I was at the Y working out with Wayne, as I do almost every day. When Wayne's next appointment showed up early, he introduced me to Vince, who was recently diagnosed with Parkinson's. He was on a search for a straight-forward book that explained and advised newly diagnosed PDers about the stark realities and the practical "what-to-dos" of Parkinson's. He'd read my exercise book, and strongly suggested that I consider writing a follow-up with a wider focus."

Vince chimes in:

"I read somewhere that silk pajamas make it easier for PD patients to move in bed? I guess that's of interest to some people. But what I wanted was the straight truth about Parkinson's from people who had actually experienced it."

What was going to change? How fast? Were there practical things I could do to make life easier? Dave had Parkinson's for thirteen years, and can obviously write, so I suggested that we team up and do a book that enlightens new PDers about what Parkinson's is really like; what you think about, how you cope, don't cope, the unexpected pitfalls, what you've learned; you know, the stuff you wish now that you'd known then."

And Chris:

"I saw a newspaper press release about a book authored by 2 Sarasota men. It was about the positive impact of exercise on Parkinson's disease, called How to Tame Parkinson's by Keeping Fit. I was diagnosed a year earlier; I'm a loyal exerciser and believe strongly in the positive impact of exercise, so I got the book and tracked Wayne down at the Sarasota Y. As soon as I met him, I knew that he was the right person for me to deal with - he was friendly, seemed very knowledgeable – his general demeanor made me feel confident."

The idea behind what he and Dave put together seemed "right on" to me. Basically, since Parkinson's is classified as a movement disorder, they concentrated on strengthening the core to improve balance. I put together a program to address the development of PD in my particular case. I also signed on with Wayne for regular therapeutic massage sessions. I'd had an occasional massage in the past at beauty spas. You can forget about that comparison. Deep Tissue Massage is a serious procedure, concentrating on areas that are stressed.

Due to high interest and good press coverage on PD, there was a new awareness that exercise, massage therapy and stretching programs were benefitting PD patients a great deal. And Wayne, Dave, Chris, and Vince were united by a common interest, and a real desire to help others by sharing their own experiences.

So here they are 4 people with the same condition that is affecting each of them differently. Common threads are a commitment to exercise, a positive attitude, a passionate desire to identify every potential way to slow or stop Parkinson's symptoms, and to help others to realize that they can have some control over their own destiny.

And, you are now reading the result of that collaboration. Since their personal experience with PD had as many differences as similarities, a questionnaire was developed to collect the information we needed from a wider group. That information was combined with personal experiences. You'll find a summary of pertinent responses from the questionnaire, along with an analysis of those responses.

In retrospect, we realize that Wayne was the catalyst, the common thread that brought the group together. Circumstances brought them to the same place; it was good fortune that they passionately agreed that one of their contributions would be to raise awareness of the critical importance of regular exercise.

What the questionnaire told us about you

u?

After a few meetings, the group realized that they needed to know still more about PD patients before beginning to write about them. And they agreed that the focus needed to be wider, to include physical, emotional, and spiritual issues.

They wanted the real story on problems and inconveniences, and every day issues that were pretty basic, not sophisticated or fancy. So, they went to the source – they developed a questionnaire for Parkinson's patients; fortunately we had a willing segment of prior participants who were enthusiastic about helping us collect the info. And, we got some powerful stories and personal thoughts to share.

More than 100 questionnaires were distributed; some were distributed at PD meetings, others were offered to patients at the doctors' office. Even though there were a few questionnaires that were not completely filled in, we collected a significant amount of information that helped us to expand our understanding and be sure we were representing a fair picture.

Our purpose in developing this unofficial survey was to gather information to help determine the needs of the existing Parkinson group, so that we could develop plans to meet those needs. It has proven to be an excellent fact-finding document for our purposes, and it may also be a useful tool for others to learn about the facts and opinions shared by this group.

Following is a copy of the questionnaire with summarized responses of the participants and annotations from the analysis. As you'll see, these summaries make it easier to compile in narrative form. And it allowed reflection on the vital personal perspective of the participants, without losing, ignoring or skipping critical information. There is some valuable quantitative data here; the surprise is the interesting and inspiring viewpoints that these people were willing to share. So here's what we found out about you.

THE QUESTIONNAIRE RESULTS

Section 1 – The Way We Were

1. What age diagnosis?
    70's = 20%
    60's = 20%
    50's = 9%
    40's = 3%

Several responders confused diagnosis date with the first appearance of symptoms, which could be years apart. Overall, it seems that Parkinson's is being diagnosed earlier

2. Any other health issues?
    Yes = 40%

(cardiac, arthritis, prostate, hypertension, cancer, high blood pressure, other)

3. How long have you had PD?
    5 yrs = 28%
    10 yrs = 10%
    20 yrs = 11%

Inconsistent methods used for determining start dates

4. Prior Symptoms?
    Yes = 48%

Tremor, gait, balance, stiffness, memory

5. First in family w/PD?
    Yes = 3 %
The great majority did not know.

6. Physically active prior to diagnosis?
    Very active = 2%
    Moderate = 41%
Later answers indicated that 27% worked out 4 to 7 days a week.

Section 2 – Getting the News

1. Initial reaction to the diagnosis
   Shock, disbelief = 31%
   Anger, sadness,-fear = 15%
   Acceptance = 7%

"God gave me 5 cards and I will play them"
"I'm afraid of the uncertainty of losing independence" "I gave up on God."

2. PD difficult to admit?
   Yes = 22%
   No = 1%

In one case, the patient did not tell anyone for 5 years. He finally told his wife when she confronted him because of his secretive behavior; she thought he was having an affair.

3. Another medical opinion?
   Who referred?
   Own Doctor = 31%
   Friend = 12%
   Research = 11%

4. Is 1st doctor still treating you?
   Yes = 29%

5. Any non-traditional treatments?
   Yes = 5%

Acupuncture, PT, stretching, Pilates, yoga, meditation

6. Looking for additional info about PD?
   Yes = 49%

7. Satisfied w/quantity & quality of info?
   Yes = 40%
   Want more info = 6   Better quality = 27%

Section 3 – What Did You Change?

1. How did you tell those closest to you?
   Spouse & closest immediately = 54%
   Waited more than a week   = 5%
   Told them personally   = 51%
   Emailed   = 2%

2. Did you join a support group?
   Yes = 28%

While a few indicated transportation problems, etc., some simply did not like support groups. "They impinge on my privacy. We learn from each other's experience, but it can be very repetitious", "Sometimes it's tough to be with those who are in the late stages of PD."

3. Would you use an email support group?
Would you use a "buddy" system, like the AA sponsor system?
   Email system = 33 yes
   Call system = 21 yes

4. Personal priorities changed?
   Yes = 36 %

"I take on one day at a time, concentrating on important 'stuff' like family and friends",
"I accentuate the positive,"
"My belief in God is restored"
"I try to spend my time 'making memories'"
"I push myself to be positive"

5. Family & friends supportive?
   Yes = 44%

6. Overwhelmed? Sorry for yourself?
   Sometime = 24%
   Never = 4%

7. Affected your sex life?
   Yes = 25%
   Sought Advice 7%

Section 4 – How Are You Doing Now?

1. What part of day do you function the best?
   - AM = 38
   - PM = 12
   - Evening = 6

"After a couple of wines! Just kidding." To divert for a moment,, it seems that alcohol may help to reduce tremor activity somewhat. Of course, there is a real concern about adding to this mix, because of the variety of medications that PD patients take. Read those labels and talk to your doctors.

2. What symptoms are most difficult to tolerate?
   - Tremors = 12%
   - Muscle soreness = 6%
   - Balance = 4%
   - Freezing = 6%

3. Does medication help to control the symptoms?
   - Yes = 48%

But this raises another issue; see the next question.

4. Impacted by side-effects?
   - Yes, various

Sleepy, sleepless, short term memory lapses, difficulty w/ sequential and/or complex problem solving

5. Relationship w/caregivers?
>Independent, owns decisions = 38%
>Need some help, mostly ok = 38%
>Dependent = 5%

It would be interesting to survey the caregivers who are in charge of these PDers to see how their answers align.

6. Temperature extremes accelerate PD effects?
>Yes = 15%

Section 5 – What Are You Doing For You?

1. Exercise?
    6 to 7 x weekly = 15%
    5 x week or less = 12%
    3 x week or less = 14%
2. Defined exercise program?
    Yes = 22%
3. Personal trainer?
    Yes = 10%
    Considering = 9%
4. Exercise focused on what?
    Core = 23%
    Balance 27%
    Flexibility – 34%
5. Aerobic activity
    Yes = 23%

What kind? ***Walking, golf, tennis, biking, swimming***

6. Exercise makes you feel good?
    Physically = 46%
    Mentally = 38%
7. Massage therapy?
    Yes = 17%
8. Stretching exercises
    Yes = 39%
9. Pro-active interest in "looking good" ***(physical appearance)***
    Yes = 39%

Take an active interest in clothes, grooming, hair dressing, and shaving – looking neat.

There is a renewed emphasis on exercise in the PD community since several authoritative studies have indicated that regular, rugged exercise has a measurable positive effect in reducing the symptoms of Parkinson. **EXERCISE IS MEDICINE** is the current slogan that many PD support groups are responding to.

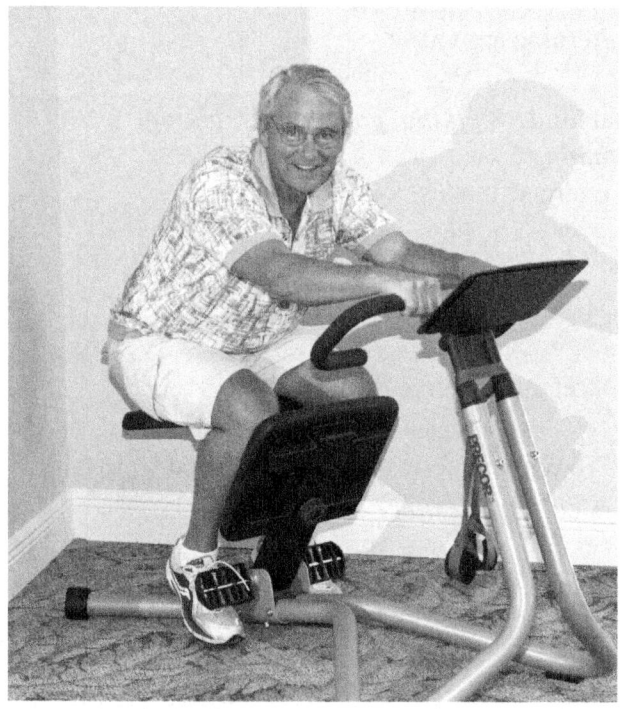

Section 6 – Where Are You Now?
Back to the Future

1. What are your major concerns/frustrations?
"The disease is progressive with no cure in sight."
Loss of mobility is a big concern.
2. Inspirational materials?
Yes = 15%
Prayer books, meditation, the Bible, Wayne Dyer, Deepak Choprah, Eckhart Tolle
3. Greatest fear?
Becoming a burden, falling, loss of mental acuity, becoming increasingly dependent.
Any positive aspects?
Newfound appreciation for life, family, friends. "I have clarified my priorities." "I realize how fortunate I am." "I work to keep my sense of humor". "This is a pain in the ass, but so is the lousy economy, inflation, war, corruption, etc. We deal with life. Period."
4. Do you follow research into PD and its potentials?
Yes = 34%
5. From where?
General news coverage and from our doctors.
6. Which research categories do you think will pay off on the investment?
A Cure? Or holding back the symptoms.
Stem cell research and gene therapy ... but when???

Thoughts on Adjusting to Your New Reality

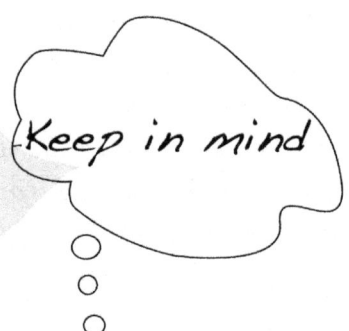

When the data from the Questionnaire was compiled and interpreted, the resulting free-form narrative provided insight into what inspires people who are destined to live in difficult circumstances, as well as the inspiration they pass on to others.

One of the early difficulties in coping with a diagnosis of Parkinson's, is dealing with the realization that you may not be able to do all that you physically were capable of before. This can weigh heavily as you learn to cope with the limitations that are now part of your new reality.

A few of you addressed that directly in the questionnaire.

"There are a lot of things I used to be good at; eg, as a nurse I was an outstanding IV starter, but no longer. I used to have a 21 handicap that was in the past. ... All of these used to weigh heavily until I adjusted to the new me. I'm now focused on keeping the new me healthy and happy. This has required a job change and new golf friends, who accept me the way I am and enjoy my company anyway.

From this experience I have learned to be cheerful, as no one wants to be around a complainer. I also work out twice a week to keep in balance."

Often people who have PD and who continue to compete in sports, sense a reduction in their physical capabilities long before an official diagnosis. Their performance begins to suffer, and they see that their games are not up to par (...pun intended). An avid tennis player says her game deteriorated from month to month. She thinks she's in the early stages of PD, but has decided to not investigate her health problems just yet. She's aware, but not ready to deal with it. She will be forced to face the reality soon enough.

And, one athlete said she lost all concentration after she first heard her doctor tell her of the diagnosis. She said she was fine, she had no questions.

"I just wanted to get out of the Doctor's office and cry".

You will see real courage in those who face the day-to-day reality of PD alone. One respondent recently lost her husband. They were very close. She fights through bouts of depression. She doesn't want to lose her independence; her kids want her to move in with them.

"I speak to the kids on the phone. I do my artwork, I go to the library, I watch movies. My greatest concern is how to plan around a progressive disease."

But the diagnosis has spurred her to commit to an aggressive exercise and weight control program. She finds that it gives her a feeling that she has some control over her body – and she has seen some improvement. We find her to be inspiring:

"Parkinson has increased my appreciation of the world around me. It has helped me to experience my recently deceased husband as being with me, and modeling for myself his courage".

We asked if there were many positive aspects of PD, most said no. A few indicated that it was just another of life's troubling issues that we have to deal with.

"Having PD demonstrates the ability to cope."

Your mood and responses were mostly balanced, however … Some pointed out that while they were concerned about their own ability to adapt to physical limitations, they recognized that those closest to them have pulled together in support; that friends cared deeply and showed compassion; that it brought them closer to God.

"I am focused more on family relationships and accomplishing all I can, when I can."

A few of you mentioned spirituality, meditation, and cited renewed interest in the Bible, and in inspirational authors like Deepak Chopra, Wayne Dyer, and Rhonda Byrne. And several have learned to pray.

All is not unrealistically rosy; the hard questions are still there and – your greatest fears were not surprising: failure to find a cure, becoming incapacitated, becoming a burden, losing mobility, and, of course, keeping your drivers' licenses. There were a few who mentioned deep and worrisome fears, with a bleak outlook and little hope.

"I took care of myself, I exercised, I ate right ... why me?"

> "Having PD demonstrates the ability to cope."

> "I am focused more on family relationships and accomplishing all I can, when I can."

> "I took care of myself, I exercised, I ate right ... why me?"

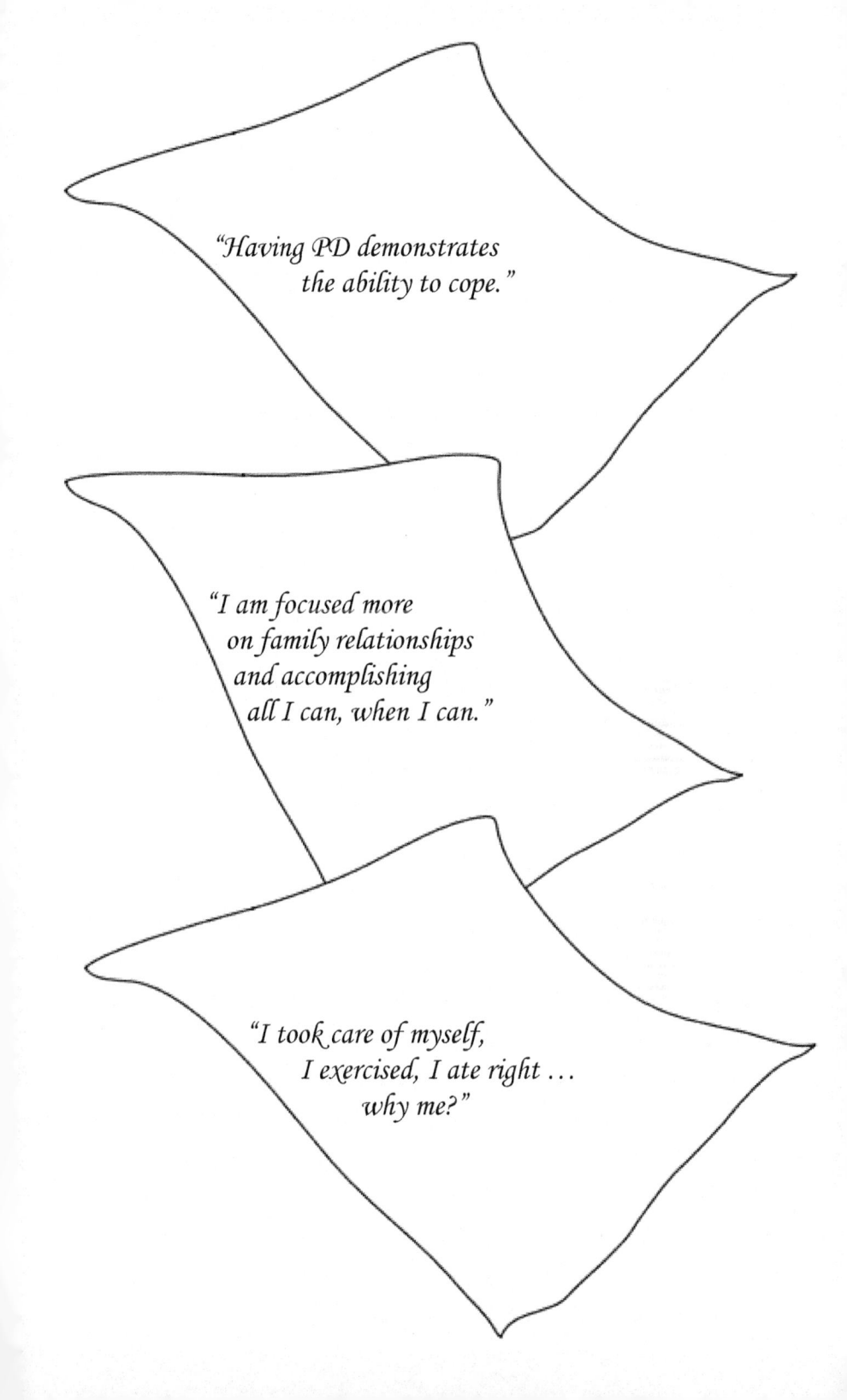

Interesting and Amusing

As you'd guess, golf and tennis are the most popular sports by far, and many who love/hate these games worried about being able to compete. Their passion for the game makes us smile –

Q. Do you participate in sports?

"Golf, if you can call it that!"

One PDer walks 18 holes 3 times a week, providing plenty of exercise. Near the end of the survey, we asked about which symptoms were the most difficult to accommodate into your everyday routine. Most responded "Tremors". But our golfer was a little more specific –

"Tremors while putting!"

A few mentioned that the most positive aspect of PD was learning to be closer to God. This contemplative thought was balanced by one participant, who listed a Handicap Parking Card as the most positive aspect.

While we enjoyed the light-hearted comments, some of the responses were more philosophical and spiritual, and brought tears to our eyes.

"It (Parkinson Disease), has been one of my greatest teachers, It has brought me closer to God, it has taught me patience with myself and others; it has taught me compassion, to myself and to others, unconditionally."

And, this participant seems grounded; and his responses reflected a practical reality. When asked his greatest fear, he responded

"None, I can handle it. Life has many surprises; I concentrate on not giving in to it." "PD is a pain in the ass. But so is the lousy economy, inflation, war, political corruption, etc. We deal with life; Period."

And, this from a good friend:

"I have a belief, since Vietnam, that for me, every day of life is a free day. With a feeling I should have died there, I live away from death, not towards it. You don't have to be a veteran to think this way. All you need is an appreciation for life as an amazing gift."

*I live away from
death, Not towards it'*

Early PD (Up to 10 Years)

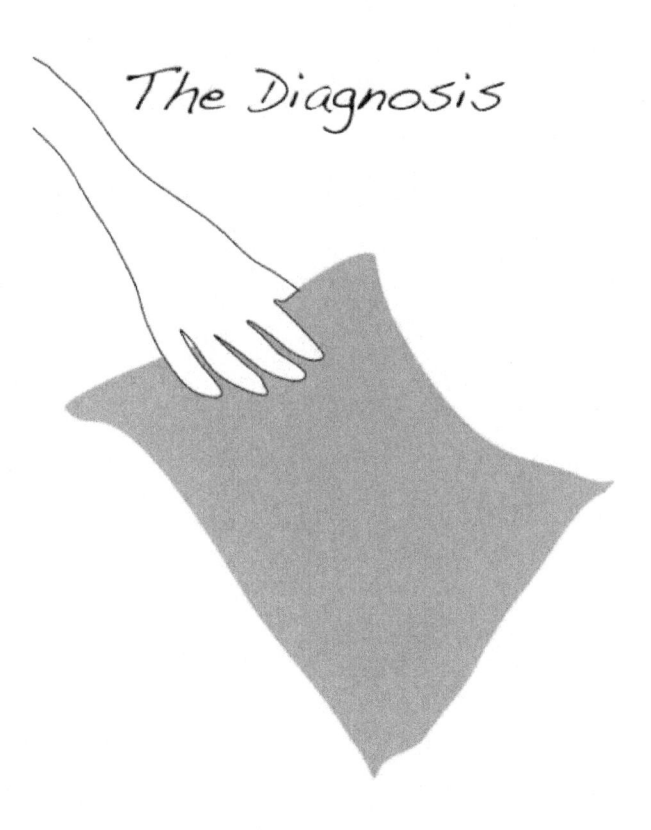

The Diagnosis

Before the official word is announced by their Neurologists, most PDers suspect that there's something significant going on. It's often tremors that appear in one hand, or both; the tremors are constant or intermittent. Their gait may change to a shuffle, and balance becomes an issue. There may be extreme fatigue, or balance problems.

There is no "formula". In other words, a few of… or some of …or all of … the above symptoms may appear intermittently, or may be obvious much of the time.

Getting "the word" officially poses a major turning point for most PDers. It affects almost every facet of their daily routines. They each vividly remember the circumstances and the cascading effect that followed.

Here's a recap of the events that followed Dave, Vince and Chris's official entry into the world of PD.

Diagnosis 1 - Dave

"Parkinson's and I have been together for over thirteen years…in a shaky relationship. A shaking left hand and a shuffling walk were my first signs, so alarmingly similar to the ones Janet Reno was experiencing at the same time, according to the media stories announcing her affliction. My immediate reaction was disbelief and total panic. "Not me!" followed by "why me?" followed by "No, I couldn't have Parkinson's!" But a visit to a neurologist confirmed that "Yes, you do have Parkinson's. Did I cry? You bet I cried, unashamedly, buckets. I decided that my life was over.

I wish that I could tell you that I faced it like a man, but I did not. I was a coward. The following months were absolute hell for me, and my family and close friends, as well. I hid from reality. I could not face the truth. I could not admit to myself or my family, or anyone else for that matter, that I had Parkinson's. I couldn't even bring myself to say the word. Was I embarrassed… ashamed…did I feel that if I didn't face it, it would go away? I was falling into a bottomless abyss of denial and despair. I was angry, frustrated, bitter, pissed…and of course I blamed God. And, I insisted on walking about with my ever-present self-created dark cloud over my head, *causing many of my friends to avoid me. I didn't blame them. I was a sorry mess.*

Fortunately I woke up, realizing that I desperately needed help. I needed to fight back, not sit back and ignore PD as it took over my life. I really needed a miracle, so I talked to the one in charge of miracles. I asked God for guidance and I believe my call was answered in many ways, including Wayne McKenna, personal trainer. His focused expertise enabled me to strengthen my physical and spiritual well-being."

*I needed to fight back,
not sit back and ignore PD
as it took over my life."*

Diagnosis 2 - Vince

You probably know that there are many differences in the type and intensity of PD symptoms that an individual exhibits, as well as differences in how fast the disease progresses, and variances in attitudes based on your basic nature.

Here's Vince:

"When I was diagnosed with Parkinson's in September of 2007, I first felt "Why me?" But then I realized there are others far worse off than I am. I made my mind up that maybe there is no cure for PD, but I could try and slow down the process. If someone says they feel sorrow for me, I simply say "Don't feel sorrow, just say a prayer". Each night I say a prayer and ask God to let me handle my PD with dignity."

Vince saw and assessed his situation logically- his attitude was "It is what it is", and he focused on problem solving and moving ahead, with minimal anger. His attitude allowed him to search for solutions and manage expectations.

Diagnosis 3 – Chris

"My job as a technology vice-president was highly visible and extremely stressful. I was in charge of the delivery and implementation of large projects for a large company. Just communicating to industry groups as well as senior management was difficult and stressful in the best of times. I had a slight tremor in my right hand for years; I used to explain it away by saying I was "jittery". It was not debilitating and not apparent most of the time.

But it became more and more pronounced. When it became hard for me to bring confidence and energy (traits that helped my success immeasurably) to the projects I was working on, I privately became concerned. The tremor seemed to be progressing at a more rapid rate and I found it to be an embarrassment.

During an annual visit to our longtime family physician, I mentioned the annoying tremor in my right arm, that it seemed to be more pronounced, and that I remembered my grandfather having one also. The doctor said that it was probably an Essential Tremor, which ran in families. He referred me to a neurologist, just "to be sure". I did not make an appointment, though, fooling myself into thinking that the condition was exacerbated by stress (which is true) and that staying relaxed was the answer. I announced to my family and friends that I had an Essential Tremor and, although I was not happy with it, I secretly was relieved that it wasn't Parkinson's. The Essential Tremor was something I could live with, because it had no other debilitating symptoms. In retrospect, what should have been obvious to all, including me, was that I was building a great case for denial that I had PD.

I saw a newspaper story about the use of Botox injections for Essential Tremor, and visited one of the Neurologists who was named in the article. The success in Essential Tremor cases was largely with head and voice tremors (a la Katherine Hepburn). The neurologist was treating only one of his patients with a hand tremor, and Botox helped somewhat. But the tremor was not on the patient's dominant side. Each treatment lasted around 3 months. Looking back, I can't believe that I went forward with the treatment – Botox works by paralyzing the muscles that contract in a tremor. That means that once I had the injections, I couldn't move or feel in certain sections of my arm and hand.. Being right-handed and having a right-handed tremor, I could barely write, and dropped at least half of what I held! The question then became, what would be worse, having a tremor or having no use of my hand. Plus, in addition to the Botox, I was prescribed some very powerful drugs *which made me extremely lethargic and made it difficult to concentrate on complex issues.*

I finally made an appointment with a neurologist – and, as he observed me walking down the hallway one time, he told me I had Parkinson's."

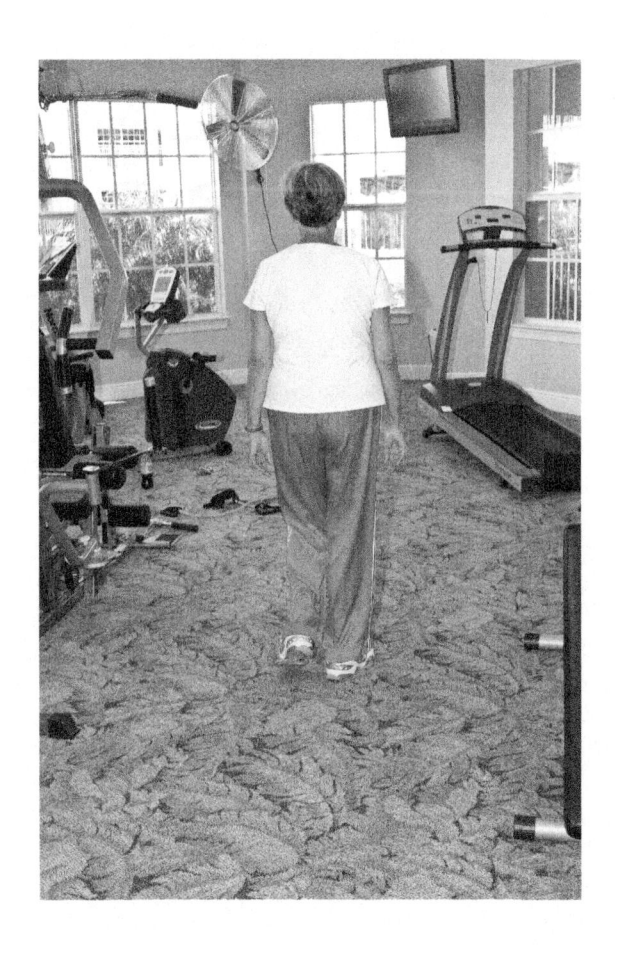

More about Dave's Diagnosis & Adjustment

"We were in London on holiday, sharing a flat with friends. One morning as we were fixing breakfast, I dropped everything I touched. It was a mess. There was cereal all over the floor and milk was flying all over the place. Later that same day, as we walked in Hyde Park, I began to shuffle and drag my feet. It was obvious to all of us that I was having some sort of a serious problem. At first my wife thought it was a stroke. I wrote it off as travel fatigue.

We were both wrong. When we got back to the US, the media was full of stories about the Attorney General Janet Reno being diagnosed with Parkinson's. I read every media story with growing fear and fury. I was experiencing some of the same symptoms; in particular, an uncontrollable tremor in my left hand. Our doctor confirmed our fears. With a sinking heart, I began living with Parkinson's in what promised to be a rocky relationship. It still is.

Meanwhile, I began to experience more symptoms, giving my negative self image more fuel to feed on. The symptoms didn't appear in set sequences either, or in degrees of severity, or on any particular schedule. It's safe to say that no 2 people have the same PD experience – it's a game of chance.

I was told that I had a "slight case" – and for 13 years, my luck held. Then, the PD began to race. The "patch" was initially part of the problem. It was designed to replace certain pills; by wearing the patch, medication would be absorbed through the skin. But in my case, it did not work, and I began to experience serious freezing, posture and balance problems, plus other symptoms, all uncontrollable until my PD medications took charge and calmed many of them down."

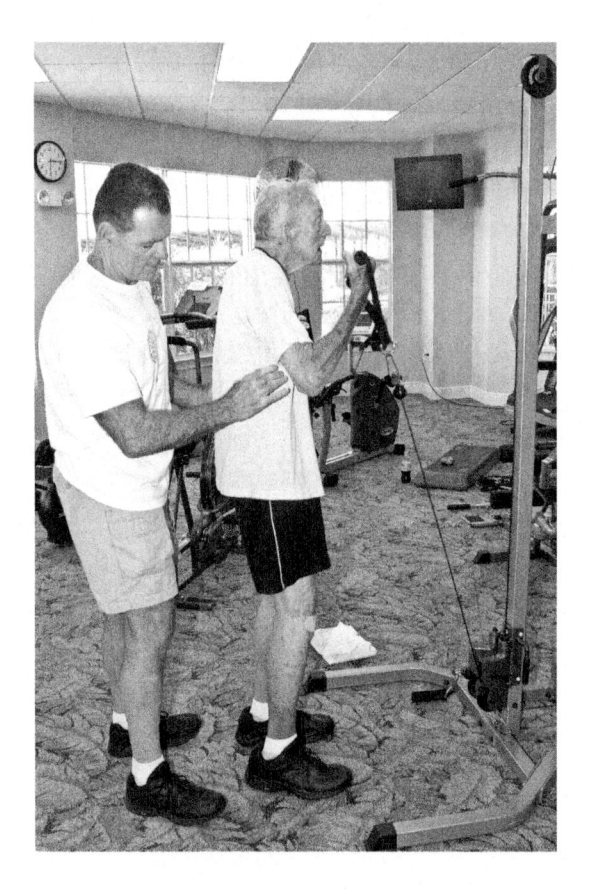

"It's safe to say that

    no 2 people have the same

        PD experience –

            It's a game of chance."

And, Chris Tries to Make Sense of it All

"I was devastated with the Parkinson's diagnosis. I'm an analytical thinker, but I couldn't find a place for this information. I was stuck, trying to approach this issue rationally, when it made no sense at all. There was no one to go to who could make it go away ... there was no one to negotiate with ... I got on the internet and, for several weeks, downloaded, read, googled... until my new doctor and my techie son told me to stop.

Aside from information overload, there was a fair amount of information that was incomplete or just plain wrong,

Of course, I told my husband about the diagnosis first, not thinking about how difficult this news would be for him. I'll keep my emotions in place and just tell you that we've been together for a long time, he is my best friend, we have many years of wonderful memories accumulated and we're still adding more. We both cried and slowly developed a plan that was largely focused on getting our real priorities straight and in order.

After logically accepting the diagnosis, it is still easy to "get stuck" and wallow in self-pity."

Chris was "stuck" until advice from the past helped her to focus on thoughts of mind over matter. Or, is it the mind that is the matter?

Chris was "stuck" until

    advice from the past

        helped her to focus on thoughts of

            "mind over matter"

                Or, is it the

                    mind that is the matter?

Reflections on Hearing the Diagnosis

"My heart sank and I didn't hear his words anymore. I tried to tune him in, but my mind was speeding along ... he was just another doctor ... I'm getting a second opinion ... he has no bedside manner ... how could he diagnose me with Parkinson's by watching me walk and touch my own nose? He's a jerk – and for my own sanity, I have to get out of here.

I was a highly compensated VP in a highly stressful environment. Although I described myself as "jittery" for years, the shaking hand increased its tempo noticeably over the past few months. After reading an article about Botox improving migraines and certain tremors, I was treated with no measurable success at all.

In retrospect, I think the low point was my friend Dawn's wedding. I realized that something had changed in me; many of my oldest and dearest friends would be there. I didn't shop for a new outfit – I didn't care.
I learned a lot about the relentless progression of PD as well as the effectiveness of the state of the art medications, which did practically stop the tremors. But the side-effects made me feel I had a carpet over my brain. My spouse, kids, grandkids, friends, all worked hard at keeping a positive atmosphere; I pretended, but really didn't care.

I started reading "head books", i.e., "The Secret", books by Deepak Chopra, Wayne Dyer – "you have the power to change anything, because you are the one who feels your feelings".

"You create your own universe as you go along."
Winston Churchill

"I discovered a book about exercise written by a local PDer and his personal trainer. Met them, developed a tough regimen that I still follow today. Sometime during this intense search for a miracle, I realized that PD wasn't the issue, I was. Physically, I had to work to strengthen core muscles and build a healthy structure; psychologically, I had to work to strengthen my psyche. It was up to me to continue to find ways to make a difference, to continue to "make memories". Damned if my mother wasn't right ... "You can do anything. You have to try ... and keep trying."

Thanks, Momma

Accepting the Diagnosis (or not) & Coping

By now, we all have developed our own ways to handle life's difficulties. Some methods work better than others, and some may be more appropriate for your personality than others. Chris has found some interesting and practical ways to "cope" (as she says, "Rhymes with hope").

"For instance, I feel that I'm fresher in the morning, so I schedule myself to do the duties that require heavier concentration and focus in the AM. This involves the consulting work I do in marketing and book editing. Stress has an immediate effect in increasing the symptoms — even positive stress.

Physically, I need to be much more aware of my environment because balance is affected, the tremor is on my right side, and it's most obvious in my right hand. The balance of medication that I'm taking now minimizes the tremor; I can often tell when I need another dose without looking at my watch, because the tremor becomes much more pronounced. I believe that the disease is progressing slowly in my case. Most of the time, I have adjusted to the symptoms. I feel that I can handle any symptom as it is now; it's very difficult though to think about how they'll be in the future — so I don't!

As my medication changes, I am now better prepared to handle side effects. Earlier, some of the effects on short term memory, concentration and problem solving capabilities really scared me. I now understand that these were the result of the medication's impact, and not dementia. So – let's see now, where was I? -what was I saying? Just kidding."

We felt a huge, and in many ways a positive, impact, much to our surprise. I take far less for granted; I'm much more aware of little things that I used to be too busy to notice. Right after the diagnosis, I was a bit depressed I think. I lost interest in things that used to be important to me – like shopping. My friends love this explanation! But, seriously, I took less interest in my appearance, which was uncharacteristic. It's tough to be sure about what the cause was, because it could have been a drug side effect. Anyway, I work hard at keeping a positive and productive attitude. I have my own secret and simple system that helps me a lot. I've identified traits that are important to me, like - Courage, Grace, Trust, Flexibility, Humor, etc. and wrote those single words on post-its. I put them in places that I use every day — on top of the TV in our bedroom, near the phone, etc. So, when I go about my daily life *and come across one of those virtues, I think about it. It's a great reminder to stay positive.*

One more observation about coping - although learning to cope is extremely important, it's not the last step in problem resolution. It is equally important to be open to change, and to be capable of adapting our behavior. Since PD is a progressive disease, we can be sure that its effects are not stagnant, so there will be multiple opportunities to learn to cope in specific situations as well as to adapt to the new environment."

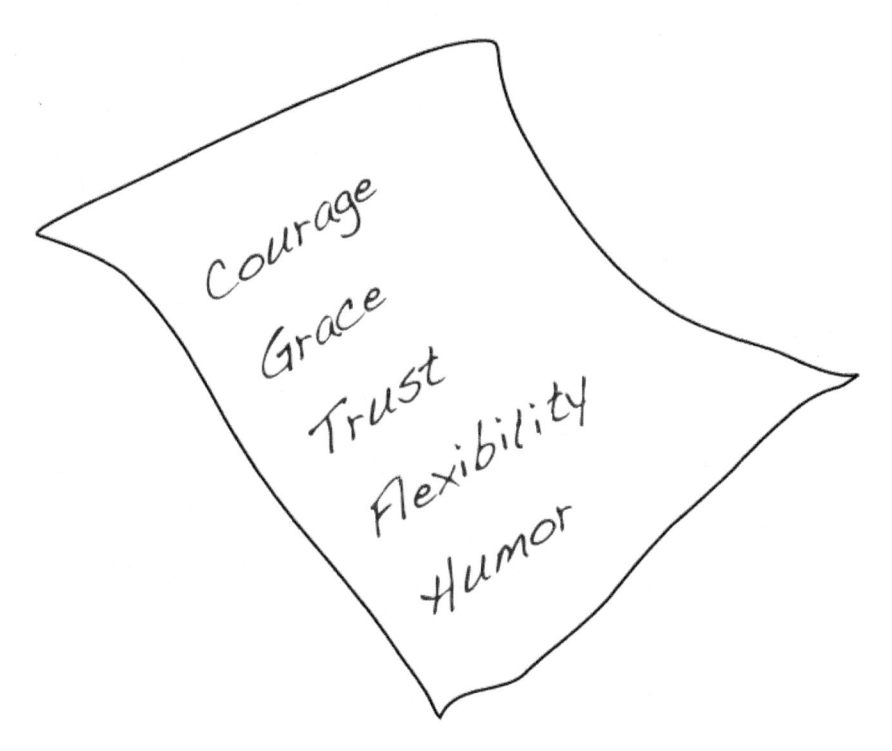

Courage
Grace
Trust
Flexibility
Humor

Mid PD (10 + years)

Caregivers

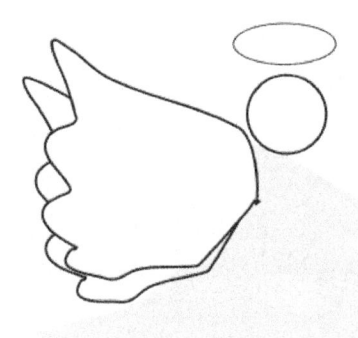

Sometimes, the person most affected by an illness is the caregiver. These kind and loving souls live day-in and day-out with their primary mission to make day-to-day life easier. They are truly angels ... Here is Sue Anderson, caregiver to Dave.

"This is a new venture for me. Being a caregiver and writing about it. My husband, Dave, has had PD for thirteen years and we thought we were lucky because his seemed like a "mild case". He was able to function well, drive his car, meet friends for lunch, type up a storm on his computer, publish a book on the benefits of exercise for PD patients, and in general carry on in his normal, tenacious, "please, Mother I'll do it myself" persona.

In the meantime, I'd been carrying on in my own creatively involved interests: first with a very intense 13-year study of watercolor painting resulting in professional status and a happy involvement in teaching watercolor. Then an all-consuming passion for designing and knitting handbags, which is still evolving hopefully into a business.

Whoa, into this picture of busy retirement and interwoven parallel lives comes the sudden change.

The monster that has been quietly lurking is suddenly making itself felt more than usual. Body tremors have begun, feet are freezing, a cane is needed, driving a car is impossible. The voice is tremulous, swallowing difficult. If there is such a thing as a PD crisis, we are in the midst of it. And it may be only just the beginning.

I'm here, I'm in it for the long run. I've awakened to the fact that the "long run" may be a lot more than I bargained for but it fortunately comes one day at a time and that's how I take it. Mother Earth? Nurse Nellie? The Pill Police? Call me what you will but I am here for you and I'll try not to baby you, smother you or belittle you. (Old parenting skills are being used here!) It helps if you are able to be tolerant of me, too. Since you no longer drive, I'll take you anywhere you need to go, just don't tell me how to get there. If I "get in your space" you need to tell me. (I know that spatial concepts are hard for you). If I misunderstand your slurred speech, be patient. Be ready for "black humor", it's one of my coping skills.

Here's a word of advice for all caregivers: carve a niche for yourself. Keep on with a hobby you care about. A wise teacher told me "you will have your art to sustain you"

It is very true. I may not paint as much as I once did, but I know it's there. Now I knit, and I have projects underway constantly. It's my reward at the end of a selfless day. I welcome input from other caregivers. We're all in this together! "

The Accidental Caregiver

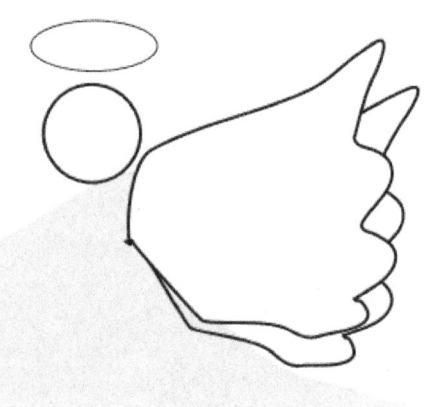

One of the most daunting tasks in providing support from outside the family for a loved one with PD is to find the right person; someone qualified professionally, and perhaps more important, someone who is temperamentally suited.

If you need someone to care for your PDer (and you certainly will want and need to have time to yourself) you'll be glad to know that they are "out there". It takes time to find them, so it may take a while. You'll need to be persistent and to know which of the support activities is most important. The likelihood of one person having all of the background and experience that you want on day 1 is low. So, prioritize that list and get the word out. Be sure that you clearly and carefully review the details of your expectations with the interviewees. Here's a good news story from a professional caregiver.

"Miracles happen" says Penny, and she absolutely believes it. She is a short, attractive, sturdy woman, and looks a decade younger than she really is. Through a series of coincidences, she is now a professional caregiver – a rare commodity in today's marketplace – and she loves her job.

She retired as President and CEO of the Business & Professional Women's Club, an organization that grew naturally as the first wave of women's executives joined the ranks of the retired. They were the first to achieve just about every new accomplishment that their gender claimed in the fight for women's rights. Some of them were good friends – although they were executives in a variety of businesses, they got to know and respect each other over the years. They were an educated, curious and relatively healthy group, and so were very active socially.

Since Penny was among the youngest, she often organized activities and outings, and provided transportation. The group was informal, but grew from a few friends to as many as 11 people. And, as the aging process did take place, their needs frequently put Penny's time at a premium. Penny's role, although centered on support and organizing, differed from a home health aide, for instance. She took additional training in order to become certified by the state of Florida, and continues to attend various health care seminars, including several for hospice care. She has a network of people who she has worked with over the years, who are trained, reliable, and empathetic. She is very much in demand. She takes on only new assignments when she thinks she and the patient can develop a relationship. She wants to be in places where she can add value; she insists that they all do physical as well as mental exercises. One of her patients who was an old movie buff, had a collection of old movies that he enjoyed watching time and again. He unfortunately lost his sight. Penny insisted that they continue to watch the movies. "What the heck – he knows them all by heart anyway." Penny thinks it actually increased their appreciation for the films in some cases, because they paid closer attention and listened more carefully.

Penny is perfectly suited for the work that she does. Whether the disease is PD, or MS, or Alzheimer's, she helps make miracles. She just got some new business cards, that say – "Quality of Life Organizer" which is a fine description of what she does. I've talked her into adding "Hope Giver", which I think, captures the essence of what she does.

Shopping List

Milk

Eggs

Hope

Optimism

We have lots of company

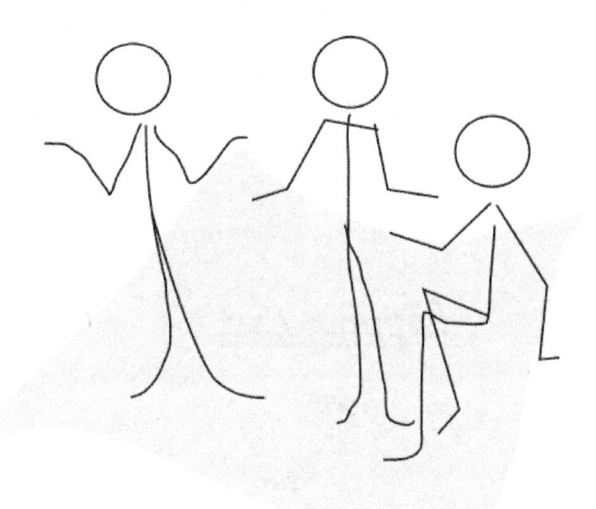

You will find that we have lots of company with "movement disorders". Here is a memoir from someone with MS. Maureen has been an inspiration as well as an example of courage and humor. But most impressive is her commitment to find a way to eke every bit of adventure out of whatever situation she was in.

"January 13th, 1996 - a "significant defining moment" in my life. I was 41 at the time. I was diagnosed with Multiple Sclerosis after just one week of really bizarre sensations in my feet. In a way, my life was jolted to a stop as the shock set in and the zillion questions swirled in my head and kept me as nervous as ever. It was SCARY. I thought I was going to be in a wheelchair forever and the more I read about MS, the more petrified I became. My head was filling up with misconceptions and I feared the future...big time.

I was a fashion designer in NYC and had been working for large accessory companies for nearly 20 years. I traveled the world for business creating products and overseeing the manufacture of them in the various countries they were produced in. My life was hectic, demanding, stressful, thrilling and exhausting all at the same time. I knew no other way. I did not love that much business travel but I had no intention of stopping. My husband was also working hard and traveling plenty so we met up on weekends somewhere we could both get a quick couple of days together. It sounded glamorous to others and sometimes to ourselves but mostly was hard work. The reality was that I was not completely happy....or healthy.

On that dreary day-Jan. 13th, 1996, the neurologist had MRI films up on the wall and was explaining to my husband and me where all the delineations were and how many "holes I had" in my brain. I remember just looking at the film and checking to see if it really was MY NAME on the film and determine if he was really talking about me. My husband listened and I was so thankful to have him with me to hear. I heard one thing: most people do not die from MS. Their life is much harder but very rarely will anyone die of MS. I decided on the spot that if I am not going to die from MS, I better do all the things in life NOW before I am in a wheelchair! I told my husband after the appt. that we must go on our postponed business trips that day. We took 2 copies of the book the doctor had about MS, got us to the airport-me crying the whole way and got on our planes to our work. I cried the entire flight while reading the book through my tears. If I wasn't dying, I better keep living......like I always had. That weekend we went skiing because I could! We hiked, we traveled more, we worked lots more.

The whole time, my bizarre symptoms continued and I let nobody know. None of my symptoms "showed". For two years I had many different episodes of MS attacks: tingling in my legs and arms, dizziness, blurred vision, etc.

On April 15th, 1997, the FDA approved a drug for relapsing/remitting multiple sclerosis that I began taking daily. It is a subcutaneous injectable drug and the doctor recommended I give it a try. So, I have taken Copaxone since its approval in the USA. It seems to be working pretty well for me, as we continue to monitor its effects, as well as the disease's progress that I have had no significant relapses in approximately 11 years. For me, it's been a miracle drug.

I am far more relaxed and feel far healthier. Recently my neurologist actually said out loud that I may never have another relapse! He said "just stay on the drug".

I look at life from a completely different viewpoint from the "me" prior to that defining day. I have spent countless time slowing down and truly enjoying life. Hopefully, I will not need that wheelchair. I take each day as a gift and feel lucky to have had the jolt of my diagnosis to enable me a more relaxed and fulfilling life."

You've Got to Accentuate the Positive

Along with a completed Questionnaire was a note written by Bonnie. We were quite impressed by her enthusiasm. Her message was filled with optimism and positive vibes. So, we gave her a call – and had a lovely chat!

"I was a nurse, and at age 50 I noticed a tremor in left small finger at rest. Then it progressed to left hand and left leg when I lay in bed at night. Of course, being a nurse I felt I maybe had a brain tumor.

After much testing, PD was diagnosed. She wasn't shocked. She thought she might have it, but hearing the diagnosis made it real. "I made up my mind that if I did have it, I was not going to let it affect my life, as long as I could fight it. It was not going to get me down. I worked with Psychiatry patients and doctors every day." ... "I was lucky, I was active, and I worked 2 jobs, and did many 16 hour shifts". "But I never got tired or depressed.

I had not water skied for 4 or 5 years so I decided that was one of my goals. Not only did I ski, I skied on one ski!. I continued that until I was 58."

One of Bonnie's doctors suspected a potential link to pesticides or well-water. She did drink from a well that was full of minerals and lots of iron. There was an iron filter on it but the water still tasted of minerals. Her ex-husband (they divorced in 1973, but maintained contact with each other) developed PD 4 years after she did. His PD progressed rapidly. His lifestyle did not include much physical activity.. At the time of the interview, his condition was deteriorating. Bonnie, on the other hand, is totally committed to regular physical training as well as a very active life-style.

"So, I strongly feel that I am in good shape because I refuse to get worse and I stay very active. Walking daily, attending a gym program 3 days a week to work out and maintain muscle control. So activity and a positive state of mind, I feel is so important. Attitude is important with any disease, I refuse to ever give up or give in to my disease. In fact I don't think about it very often. I ignore it."

Now this next bit of info makes me smile every time I read it!

"I have moved to Tennessee with my sweetheart from 1958 who I had not seen for over 46 years. He has to be a little crazy because his deceased wife had Alzheimer's for over 10 years before she died and now he has me with Parkinson's. He says no he's not crazy, just in love. So I am having a wonderful life."

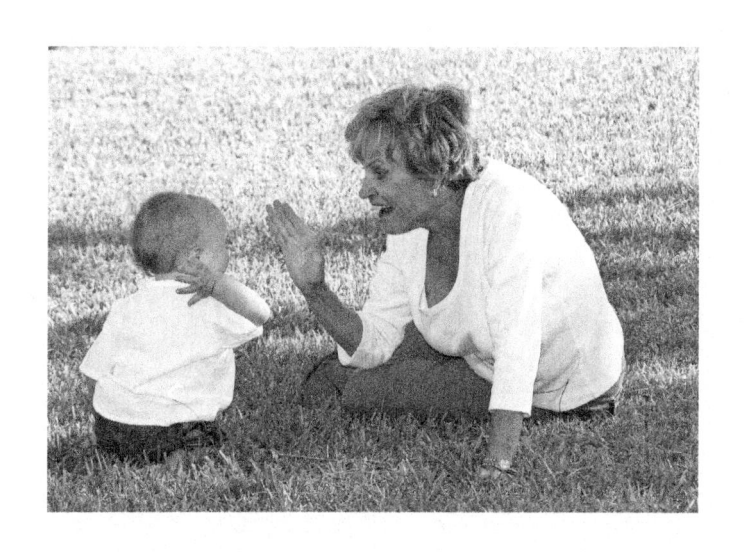

Eliminate the Negative!

As we worked together on the format of the book, our kind, generous and talented graphic artist, Sherry talked about her cousin, Hazel.

"She is such an inspiration. She believes that there's nothing she can't do – and you know, she's right. She was operating a new business when she was diagnosed with Parkinson. She's so unwavering and single-minded that she accomplishes just about anything she sets out to do. Not because she's superhuman, but because she's determined. You should really talk to her."

And, so we did. Early in the conversation, we wondered if there was any one thing that she attributed success to.

"I'm lucky in a lot of ways; and being a natural optimist gives me an edge in dealing with life's little surprises. I believe that "It is what it is" and we have to deal and cope with whatever life brings us.

And, I was lucky enough to have my father as an example in my life. What a guy he was! His optimism and good humor helped to shape the way I looked at life."

She's always been a good and adventuresome cook. Her salad dressings were "fabulous;" and more and more people began asking her to make some as take-out. After the kids were grown, her daughter talked her into trying to build a business of her own.

"I began selling my bottled dressing at a local craft festival. It was a successful start, even though I didn't have any real business background. What I did have was plenty of support and confidence that I could make it. I absolutely believed in myself and in the dream. There was no "Plan B" for me. Plan B means that you think there's a chance that Plan A will fail.

Looking back, I can see that what was really telling was my very first venture as a budding entrepreneur at the age of 12. My cousin Sherry and I were at the beach house and wanted to make some money. There were no jobs – we decided to make and deliver baked goods. We were thrilled to have sold whatever we made. We were also surprised to find out that we had to pay my aunt back for her initial investment in our business, and that we also had to allocate money for new supplies. Business 101 as pre-teens!"

She now carries 8 dressing flavors: poppy seed, sugar free poppy seed, balsamic vinaigrette, honey cinnamon, rosemary lemon, herb garden, buttermilk dill, and ginger lime. The dressings are available locally in and near Knoxville, Chattanooga and Asheville.

As far as Parkinson is concerned, when she got the diagnosis she was angry- it seemed so unfair. But, she soon developed a rigorous exercise program, in the belief that a healthy and strong body will slow the progress of the disease.

"At the least, it gives me the feeling that I have some control over my fate. I have a lot of life to live and this is not going to stop me!"

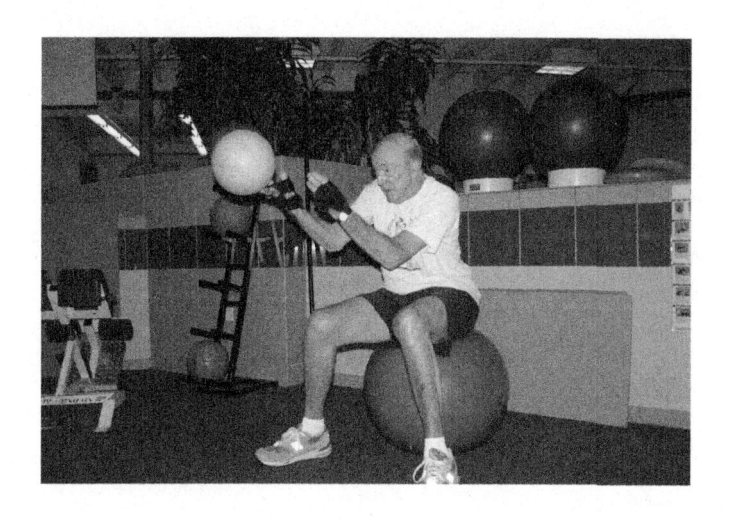

Exercise is medicine!

That was one of the enduring messages that stayed with most of the attendees of this year's Parkinson Symposium. Our group has been totally convinced since day one that rigorous and frequent exercise not only slows that progress of PD, it actually wipes out some of the symptoms. Up until recently, it wasn't easy to get verifiable data on this proposition; clinical studies are expensive and researchers are onto more exotic experiments.

But, if exercise is medicine, who writes the prescription?

Dave Anderson was ahead of his time. After working out a program under Wayne's direction, specifically to address Dave's symptoms, Dave and Wayne's assignment presented itself when they decided to write a book, a basic self-help primer to share what was learned. The result was <u>How to Tame Parkinson's by Keeping Fit, My Total Commitment + The Right Personal Trainer</u>, which targets not only those with PD, but also their caregivers, families and friends.

"These specialized routines are customized to help confront Parkinson's, physically and mentally. There's nothing exotic here – There are a lot of crunches; many, many crunches. But the sheer number and combinations provide focus on your

"core" and on balance. It also provides a hard-hitting strategy that counter- attacks on the battlefields where Parkinson's fights diligently to take over -- balance, mobility, posture, speech, depression, to name a few.

While working with Wayne I realized that he was a deep-thinker, a man who took life very seriously, and believed in God. We often discuss spiritual and inspirational subjects. While working to strengthen our bodies, we found help and inspiration to build our spiritual support foundations.

How do you do Dr. Wayne Dyer, Joel Osteen, Rhonda Byrne? No matter how many times I hear your inspirational messages, I learn something new."

*"Your messages fill my heart
with hope
and optimism."*

Later PD

We Got the Message

We heard about a study that was conducted in the mid-west that indicated in preliminary results that vigorous, regular exercise substantially reduces the progress of PD. Some participants said that they believed their disease had stopped progressing. Chris is a strong proponent of exercise as medicine:

"You may remember that Dale and I are joggers and exercised regularly, and we still do. We were able to put together a program focused on "core" muscles and balance. I even went to a "stretch man" who specializes in a program that focuses on stretching as an important component of an exercise program.

So now, we are evangelical about spreading the message – exercise every single day, no excuses. I spend about an hour doing the mat core exercises I mentioned above.

And, at least 3 times a week, with few exceptions, I either walk / run 3 miles (slowly, to be sure), or spend 45 minutes on the elliptical trainer."

Putting together an individualized program for each client, is an important initial step for a seasoned personal trainer. The assessment should begin as you are saying hello. We were unaware at first, but as we got to know Wayne, we realized that he watches your every move, and notes your posture, stance, steadiness, etc., and uses all the information he collects, when putting together your program.

"If a client is unable to accomplish a certain exercise I feel is necessary, I simply plug in a more user-friendly one that will work on strengthening and toning the target muscles without undue stress. That's one reason why I prefer to train in a fully equipped fitness center that offers a choice of equipment and facilities."

Once you can complete a session on your own, you can integrate it into your own schedule; many people do not need a personal trainer on a continual basis. They continue solo, and if conditions change, they meet with a personal trainer to adjust their routines.

It is sometimes discouraging to work so diligently on strength, posture, balance, and hit a bump in the road ... sometimes it's necessary to rebuild the drills to match abilities. Sometimes they need to be simplified sometimes they need to be more challenging. What is a constant necessity is the availability of a trained advisor to monitor progress and further customize routines.

Take these comments as guidelines when you look for the right personal trainer. You don't need to look for a new best friend, but you do want to be sure that you review qualifications and look for one who has the right skills, professional training and who can successfully deal with PDers.

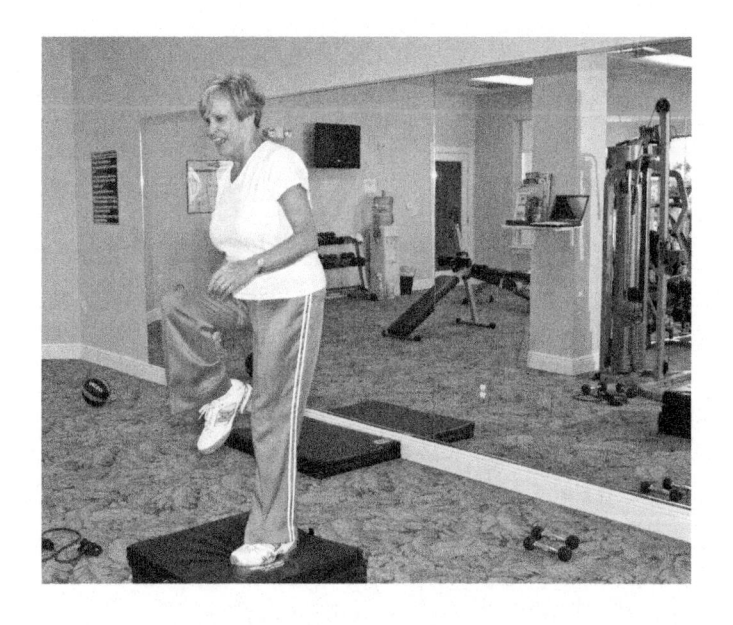

Good Bye Wheels - By Dave Anderson

This is one of the most controversial and emotional issues brought to light in our survey!

"First, I voluntarily gave up driving my car at night. Next I realized that my reaction time was becoming slower in my day driving. It was no longer, would I give up driving? It was when would I give it up. It was an extremely difficult decision to make, but ultimately, I knew it was time to do it. The "quit while you're ahead" motto whirled through my head, making more and more good sense. So I bit the proverbial bullet, and marched into the motor vehicles office and voluntarily became a non-driver. The 'better safe than sorry" pitch to other PDers in the same boat is my editorial in this one.

Remember that heady feeling the first time your Dad let you slip behind the wheel of the family car? There was no driver ed in those days. It was up to your Dad, Mom or older sibling, to teach you to drive. It was especially exciting for me, because we were in the middle of WWII, when the one and only family car was a pre-war model, all black, with window wings rather than 'air', and running boards and roomy front fenders ideal to ride on. Gas and tires were rationed (if available, and then only if you had enough ration stamps).

Impromptu family rides were considered the height of luxury. When Dad could save enough gas, the entire family would pile in for a ride around town with all the windows open to cool off on a hot summer's night. I was giddy with excitement and, yes, a pinch nervous, and hoping that my friend Willard who lived across the street was watching, consumed with envy as he saw me climb in the driver's side.

Where am I going with this remembrance? That all good things come to an end! Here am I, sixty-plus years later, once again without a license to drive a car.
It began with a routine notice from the state Motor Vehicles Department, reminding me to renew my driver's license before my next birthday.

I'd been driving with no serious problems during my thirteen-plus years with PD.

In fact, I've been driving safely with only a few of the usual minor incidents (not including the NH deer that leaped over a stone wall and made mincemeat of my Camry's front end) since I passed my first driver's test over sixty years ago. My Dad was a careful man, thus he taught me to always take my driving seriously, which I practiced throughout my many years of safe driving through most of the USA, plus bits and pieces of Canada, the UK and Germany's notorious speedway, the Autobahn.

I may have been able to have a few more months behind the wheel, but my PD was nudging me with new surprises, and I noticed my response time was slowing down. I was concerned, and yes, disappointed. So far I'd been spared the "double vision" that some PDers complained about; mostly as a result of medications.

But, the reality was that it would have been a shame, after all of this angst and drama, to be involved in an accident. We knew what the issues are – we were just at the difficult decision time! Result, I bit the proverbial bullet, marched into the motor vehicles office and voluntarily became a non-driver. Ta-dum!!!

That was the easy part. Being without wheels takes serious life adjustments. I sorely miss the spontaneity that driving offers. I can no longer hop into my Camry and fire off to wherever, whenever I please. I've become dependent on others to ferry me to and from my daily activities, appointments and errands, meaning that from now on I'm a hitchhiker. This will take some getting used to, and require patience.

Did I give Auld Lang Syne a game try when I drove for the last time? Was I sad? Teary? Did I have bittersweet thoughts and memories? No. Actually I was perplexed, thinking about how unbelievable my future would be without driving. I would never again sit behind the wheel of a car. But before I reached the end of the line, I relaxed, undoubtedly hummed a nameless tune, and simply enjoyed my last ride behind the wheel. So, some of my precious personal independence has gone with my wheels. And, I know it's not over and that I have yet to realize the full impact of the results. But I'm proud of myself for following my good sense rather than my ego, and making the right decision at the right time."

Striking the Right Balance

By Dave Anderson

"I was nervous as I arrived at the YMCA fitness center for my scheduled workout with Wayne. Our session wasn't my concern. After nearly a decade of working with this charismatic personal trainer, I knew I could count on the usual fine-tuned and challenging session. Wayne was always prepared, no matter what my Parkinson's was dishing out.

What worried me that day was that I felt strangely wobbly and unsure of my balance. This new and unwelcome PD symptom had begun so abruptly, along with occasional terrifying falls that was difficult to stop once under way."

(A word about PD-induced falls. Think of the first time you put on a pair of roller skates and tried to stand up - weeeeeeeeee. You were suddenly out of control, and your balance turned rubbery, and you were headed for a fall, right? But, remember how you practiced, and hung on to a friend or a railing, until you ultimately learned to control your balance, and enjoy yourself? It took diligence and practice, but you were soon able to control your body's balance, and take fewer falls. It's the same with PD.)

As every PD veteran knows all too well, the disease progresses at unpredictable rates, making us fearful of which motor skills will go next, and when. And 'go' they do, without any warning.

"I had lived with a relatively 'light' case of Parkinson's for thirteen years, and was hopeful that I'd missed the more serious debilitating and unwelcome 'surprises' of the disease. Alas, it wasn't to be.

My advanced PD began not long after the new 'patch' was prescribed. It did not improve or eliminate my PD symptoms; they seemed to accelerate. I experienced freezing (a feeling not unlike having both feet stuck firmly to the floor, unable to lift or move) for the first frightening time, which short circuited my balance and gave me a preview of the falls to come. I stopped using the patch before it was withdrawn from the market with absolutely no explanation. But that didn't help me. My symptoms, old and new, were moving ahead at a faster pace."

(An important note about keeping track of your PD action: PD medicines react differently on different PDers. That's why it's a good plan to keep an informal daily log -- in a notebook or on a PC file -- noting any and all reactions, symptoms, concerns, movements, etc., ready to discuss with your doctor at your next visit, if it can wait. Some reactions require immediate advice from your doctor. Don't change dosage or stop taking medications without your doctor's advice, and be sure to communicate with him thoroughly and regularly.)

"With my PD still accelerating, I was thankful that I'd stuck with Wayne. I could reap the obvious advantages of working with this seasoned personal trainer who specializes in movement disorders, who continually updates his training skills and techniques, and who takes a personal interest in his clients and their needs. Where would I be today if I had already discontinued working with him? Up the proverbial creek without a paddle, that's where! Instead, I've gained a good friend and a priceless teammate!

And again to my benefit, he learns from my symptoms - he appraised my iffy balance situation, and methodically re-planned my workout, factoring in the basic balance enhancing drills necessary to help rebuild confidence in my balance. His initially scheduled strength building session for that day would keep until next time. That day he knew that I needed specialized help."

"C'mon, Dave, let's play ball!"

"Out on the gym floor we walked, and began tossing the basketball back and forth, as we walked parallel across the floor. Slowly my

confidence began to recharge as I concentrated on catching and throwing the ball back and forth. I almost forgot about my nervousness and fear of falling, as we continued tossing the basketball. Once I was noticeably relaxing, Wayne switched to kickball using a small yellow balance ball, similar to soccer, which I immediately got in to, forgetting my balance and fall fears."

Wayne's 'impromptu' workout is included for your information and use.

It's interesting to note that restoring confidence is critically important when we encounter new problems – more important in some situations than the limitation itself.

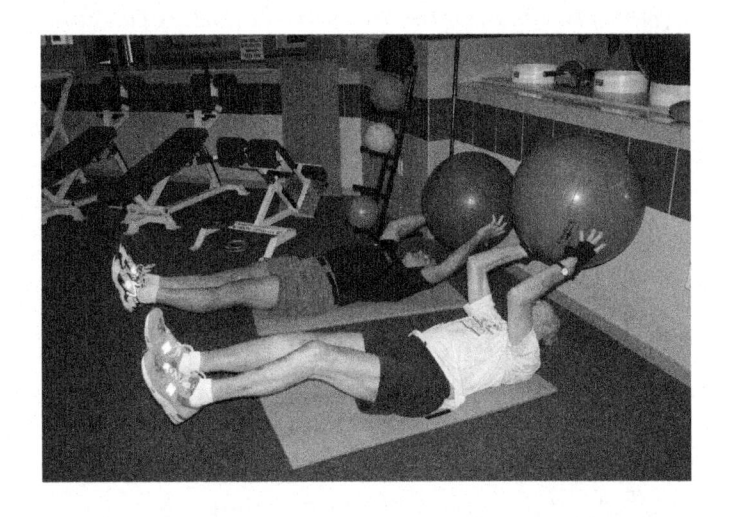

Impromptu Gym Drill Workout

for Balance Control

- Basketball toss: walk parallel, toss ball to partner with outer arm, reverse and change arm
- Basketball throw: facing wall throw ball underhand, overhand, from chest
- Kickball: played soccer style with a small yellow balance ball, or a basketball once comfortable with movements.
- Square drill: using a marked gym floor square, move sideways, shuffle, backwards, forwards, diagonal, repeat & mix, until movement and balance control become natural, more comfortable

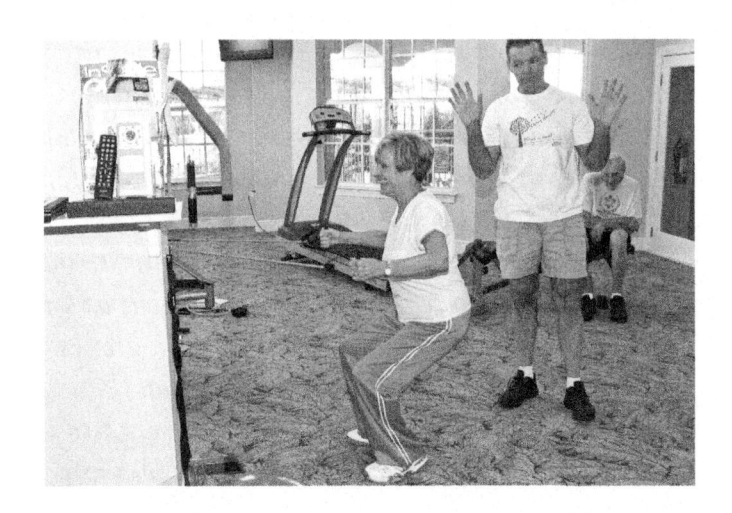

What Now? - Dave

After Dave's scary experience with increased symptoms as well as new ones, he continues to focus his energy on recording his experiences and feelings for the PD community. He does a great job here in discussing his fears as well as his inspirations.

There are several PD related issues that you will probably encounter to some degree, and although they are mentioned in most PD literature and are not major physical surprises, they can cause as much or more inconvenience and disruption to daily life. Dave addresses these, beginning with Speech, Handwriting and Memory.

"Speech difficulty announced itself (pun!) with stuttering and slurring, as well as a much softer voice. It was obvious that I was difficult to understand; sometimes I'm sure I sounded drunk. It's embarrassing to see frustrated people get that "what the hell is this guy saying?" look. My Neurologist recommended a speech therapist, and I am beginning to see and hear improvement as long as I continue to work routinely on the exercises. My handwriting is indecipherable. It has deteriorated from a passable, readable script to "chicken tracks". "Memory loses its edge, short term, in particular. Fortunately this is often a

side-effect to medication, particularly Parkinson meds.

If you were to ask me what I considered my most difficult challenge precipitated by PD, my immediate answer is loss of freedom. The why is simple – I can no longer come and go as I please, when I please, where I please. Since voluntarily giving up my driver's license when I realized my reaction time was becoming dangerously slow, I've had a difficult time coping with the resulting loss of freedom. I sometimes feel trapped and even imprisoned. No longer can I hop into the Camry and drive to the Y any time I please, meet the guys for a coffee or nosh, go off by myself exploring, or wandering, or shopping, listening to Wayne Dyer most of the time.

Now, I have to depend on family and friends for transportation, which boils down to my "scheduled" activities. Frivolous trips are few and far between, as are spontaneous "jaunts". I know folks want to help out, but they have their own "musts" and responsibilities, and I appreciate what they're able to do for me. I will continue to look for innovative ways to be able to get around easier. I've "graduated" to a walker, so taking me out means hefting, folding, unfolding. It's just another added stress.

This brings me to the second stage of my most difficult challenges precipitated by PD - loneliness, the out-of-sight, out-of-mind stage that could hit me in the future; a time when I may be less mobile and unable to get to the Y to work-out and socialize, or anywhere else for that matter. This thought terrifies me. I'm a people person and I need to be around people. For this reason, I am learning to take one day at a time to accomplish and enjoy. And each day I thank God for my blessings, and for his guidance, and I challenge Him for a cure to this destructive disease.

I believe that because of my rigorous and demanding physical exercise regimen & working with a pro like Wayne I have been able to slow down my PD progress but not stop it, as evidenced by my now necessary tri-wheeled walker, and portable wheel chair. to use when "freezing" acts up And, because PD forced me to look inwardly and has focused me on becoming increasingly spiritual, I am evolving into a kinder, more caring person, a person who even I began to like once again.

We confirm every day the realization that regular, rigorous physical exercise is essential to dealing with PD. We also confirm that attitude, positive attitude, is just as important. You are in control and you have the ability and the tools to increase both... do it!

Rediscovering faith had a lot to do with this transformation. During our exercise sessions, we often talk about God's will, our purpose in life, and the mysterious ways He directs us. I believe that his mission for me is to help others, as I've been helped. I get great fulfillment in helping others who are in a similar situation, and want someone to talk to – a kind of informal counseling. We talk about how I shook off the "why me" feeling, how to deal with concerns about mental capabilities, and many other facets that only someone who has experienced the disease can relate to.

I am so fortunate to have a home based "cheering squad." My wife and daughter are always there with love and support; they enable me to achieve physically and to keep me balanced, in several different ways. The longer I work in this way, the more I learn about myself and how to concentrate my efforts on helping others. This personal transformation has been among the most meaningful events in my life."

What Now? – Chris

Chris was pleased, but a bit nervous when her doctor agreed that she would be a good candidate for DBS. Since there were several criteria that DBS candidates had to meet, she planned to go through the testing procedure while making a final decision. She decided that there was no point in getting too involved until the basic qualifications nailed down.

"I was surprised to discover that the pre-op procedures included several hours of psychological testing which covered your memory and problem-solving abilities. There was an emphasis on what expectations you had for the outcome of DBS, which was a good thing to clarify. The most difficult part of the testing was the withdrawal from drugs during the 2 week period preceding the surgery. When the surgery date was set, I seriously thought through the implications of what we were about to do. And, I discovered more new insights about myself – first, I am more of a risk-taker than I realized, and second, I want the responsibility for decisions I make. Although I discussed the surgery with family and friends, I didn't ask for their opinions as to how to proceed. I don't want them to feel that they are somehow responsible for the outcome.

I returned home the next day after the surgery. Recovery was uneventful. But, since you are awake for part of the surgery, and because it's necessary to drill holes into the skull, I did generate a fair amount of attention.

I was up and about in a couple of days and felt better (steadier, mentally sharper, with more energy). BUT, several weeks into the recovery period, the incision did not look or feel right.

After several meetings and consultations we realized that the most prudent course of action would be to remove the device. I argued to keep it, because I was seeing noticeable improvements, and hated to give them up. . .I was feeling so good!!!

The device is out; Kaput; no mas. But, I am still noticeably improved. I am now taking nearly 30% less medication, have very high energy, less tremor, improved balance, etc. I continue to be a faithful exerciser, and will rarely pass up a chance that involves physical activity. When I went to see the surgeon for a final visit to determine if all was well from his viewpoint, he said –

Come back and see me when you look like you have Parkinson's.

A joke, of course, but one that is essentially the plan. I keep close track of changes, both physical and mental, and monitor my ability to cope in an ever-changing, more limiting environment. It's important to be aware of new obstacles and limitations, to figure out how to cope while keeping a positive attitude. Don't let it drag you down!

I still check into the progress of clinical trials that are currently being conducted, and I am doing more research to find if there are alternatives within the DBS treatment.

In reality, I would be well satisfied if I could stay in this present condition.

In the meantime, I've signed up for Tap Dancing lessons!"

In Summary

Coping ... Is that all there is?

We pointed out earlier in the book that although "learning to cope is extremely important, it is far from the last step in problem resolution. It's equally important to be open to change, and to be capable of adapting our behavior." Coping is essential, but it is passive, and it implies acceptance.

So, how do we get from here, to there? How do we enable ourselves to refresh our thinking about day-to-day issues so they don't drag us down? Once we analyze and understand the problem, the question then is, how do we take charge?

There certainly is a real challenge in living with a progressive disease that exhibits symptoms differently. You need to think about how these specific issues may affect your plans. And, a lot will depend on how much tolerance you have for uncertainty. Some of us are comfortable living with surprises, while others cannot tolerate a high level of uncertainty. But we can all learn from reading in "Movers and Shakers" about the heart-warming stories of courage and stamina, as well as tried and true ways to minimize negative impacts. If we choose to, we can learn to change, when we need to. While self-interest often gets a bad rap, we can change for our own self-interest or, to the contrary, we can choose not to change. "Don't go changin', to try to please me ….I love you just the way you are." Stevie Wonder.

Any changes that are implemented successfully can be leveraged if they are shared so that we broaden the impact of the change. Most are relatively simple and seem easy enough to adopt. Like developing an exercise regimen and then sticking to it. Because, we all know that **Exercise is Medicine**. But despite the renewed interest in this simple, but proven effective remedy; despite the availability of resources and information about exercise for PDers, it is still difficult to change our habits and lifestyle to accommodate an exercise routine.

It also can be difficult to work on the changes that affect your attitude, but those changes are just as important; they can help you to look at things more optimistically and not be overwhelmed by what you fear lies ahead. It's more than "changing your attitude." You did not choose to be depressed. Attitude is about letting yourself achieve a positive frame of mind. It's not easy. It's about taking time to empty your mind of the stresses, negative feelings, and reactions that you have accumulated, and then enabling yourself to relax and to be open to new possibilities.

First take a look at those who are in similar situations and who benefitted by making serious changes in their outlooks. By seeing what others have seen and understanding that you are not alone, you can then identify the issues that are confronting you and allow your mind to then discover the solutions that you know about. Sounds simple, but you know that sometimes it's not so easy. It takes practice and commitment, and trust in your own judgment. If you have faith that you can change the future by changing your perspective, it all becomes much simpler. In some ways, this solution is the easiest and most beneficial because all you need to do is think and have faith in the outcome.

"When you come to the edge of all the light you know and are about to step off into the darkness of the unknown, faith is knowing one of two things will happen; there will be something solid on which to stand, or you will be taught to fly!" Barbara J. Winter, Motivational Speaker.

It's a surprise to some to learn that a key to finding answers is silence. Think about the issues, close your eyes, and wait. "We become what we think about; meditation is thought power." Earl Nightingale.

What you have embarked on is a discovery process. For songwriter James Taylor the "process of discovery" is "being quiet enough and undisturbed enough for a period of time so that the thoughts can begin to sort of peek out, and you begin to have emotional experiences in a musical way." In other words you can't force discovery, simply think all your thoughts and let your mind discover a solution.

"When the voice and the vision on the inside become more profound, clearer and louder than the opinions on the outside, you've mastered your life." Dr. John Demartini. "You become what you think about most, and you attract what you think about most".

Meditation is an excellent way to put yourself in that framework. If you do not presently meditate, put "learn to meditate" at the top of your to do list. There are plenty of self-help books available, as well as CD's and DVD's. · Check out www.healthjourneys.com. There is a CD series which includes "A Meditation to Help with Parkinson's Disease." By Belleruth Naparstek.

Oprah Winfrey once said, "The greatest discovery of all time is that a person can change his future by merely changing his attitude." In other words, the greatest discovery of all is how attitude changes your life. If you believe it you know it, which is something that the father of American psychology, William James also believes. "The greatest discovery of my generation is that a human being can alter his life by altering his attitudes." As Winston Churchill once said, "You create your own universe as you go along."

You will discover that sometimes the answers are more obvious: Enrico Fermi, the physicist who built the first experimental nuclear reactor said, "There are two possible outcomes: if the result confirms the hypothesis, then you've made a measurement. If the result is contrary to the hypothesis, then you've made a discovery." Let your brain think of an alternate discovery today and you're on your way.

And as others have discovered, when the solutions are not obvious, when there are no "eureka moments," sometimes you need to break it down. Artist Chuck Close known for his massive-scale portraits, said, "If you're overwhelmed by the whole, break it down into pieces." Every big thing breaks down into lots of little things. That's where everything begins.

And there's another ingredient others have found and consider profound. For Mother Teresa, "faith in small things is where your strength lies." For Mohandas Gandhi "Strength does not come from physical capacity, but determination." For Marcus Aurelius strength is "not outside but in your mind."

Take pride in your achievements. This life is about you. If you are not already involved in sports, or art, or teaching, or any outside interest, find something you enjoy doing, something that you're good at, and want to have fun at. (Hopefully, these could be one and the same.) And look for opportunities to do it. Volunteer - Start a business - Work collaboratively - Create poetry - Write a book. (about Parkinson?)

And take the time to evaluate your work. Listen to others, to their critiques and their praise. "Encouragement is oxygen for the soul."

"Correction does much, but encouragement does more."Johann Wolfgang Goethe.

When you've become involved and passionate about your involvement, you'll find that life becomes much easier all around. You'll have more friends and opportunities, because you are more interesting. You'll see the positive impact you are actually making. You'll also see positive reactions from those around you…you'll be on the right path!

Because… "There are only 2 ways to live your life. One is as though nothing is a miracle. The other is as though everything is a miracle." Albert Einstein.

And, what we make of it, despite the obstacles, is the real miracle!

Acknowledgments

A couple of specific acknowledgements:

Sue Anderson provided support, both physical (many delicious casseroles to sustain us during meetings) as well as consistent moral support through many discussions to help us to understand the unique pressures on the Care Givers.

Wayne McKenna has from the beginning represented the view that exercise is medicine. He truly embodies the message by helping us to commit to reasonable programs that are adaptable to our unique life styles. He and Vince Doherty provided early on-going input and a steady influence. Vince's view of the world provided a fresh look to our discussions. His recognition of what a newly diagnosed PDer needed helped us formulate the content.

While Chuck Snyder and Redente Picazio provided rigorous reviews and asked the hard questions, they managed to lace their critiques with encouraging words that left us confident and committed. And Chrissie Ludwig took on the final editing with the same attention to detail that she does in most endeavors, and still remembered that encouragement is good for the soul.

And, to Sherry Erb– this entire effort would have been far less successful, and far less fun, without her wonderful and imaginative illustrations. We loved working with you, and with Lynne Fales whose technical help and incredible patience kept us on track!

And, to Dr. Sutherland and the professionals on his team, who helped us find the right answers, our thanks for also asking the right questions.

And Dale Ludwig and Sue Anderson, our heartfelt appreciation for all you do each and every day, particularly keeping upbeat and optimistic. You are the most impacted by our Parkinson's; you bear the burden of not only supporting us day-to-day, but also of witnessing the slow progression of PD.

And kids and grandkids play a much larger role than they would believe, providing joy and diversion, and helping us to not dwell on our "condition". They are wonderfully irreverent.

And, we are blessed to have a wonderful group of friends, who we have shared most our lives with. We are so lucky to have been able to keep these witty, smart, helpful, compassionate, people as part of our lives for nearly 40 years. Their influence and endless humor helps every one of us as we traverse this rocky road. Thank you. And, thank you, Ben Arbuckle.

Thank You!

PD Notes

PD Notes

Date:_____

Meeting with: _____

Contact info:

_____
_____
_____

Cell: _____

E-Mail:_____

Medical / technical
info:_____

_____
_____

General Observations / Follow up:

_____
_____
_____

Thoughts /observations to inspire:

_____
_____
_____

- PD Notes

Date:_____

Meeting with: _____

Contact info:
_____
_____
_____

Cell: _____

E-Mail:_____

Medical / technical info:_____
_____
_____

General Observations / Follow up:
_____
_____
_____

Thoughts /observations to inspire:
_____
_____
_____

- PD Notes

Date:_____

Meeting with:_____

Contact info:
_____
_____
_____

Cell:_____

E-Mail:_____

Medical / technical
info:_____
_____
_____

General Observations / Follow up:
_____
_____
_____

Thoughts /observations to inspire:
_____
_____
_____

- PD Notes

Date: _____

Meeting with: _____

Contact info:
_____
_____
_____

Cell: _____

E-Mail: _____

Medical / technical info: _____
_____
_____

General Observations / Follow up:
_____
_____
_____

Thoughts /observations to inspire:
_____
_____
_____

- PD Notes

Date:_____

Meeting with: _____

Contact info:
_____
_____
_____

Cell: _____

E-Mail:_____

Medical / technical
info:_____
_____
_____

General Observations / Follow up:
_____
_____
_____

Thoughts /observations to inspire:
_____
_____
_____

- PD Notes

Date:_____

Meeting with: _____

Contact info:
_____
_____
_____

Cell: _____

E-Mail:_____

Medical / technical
info:_____
_____
_____

General Observations / Follow up:
_____
_____
_____

Thoughts /observations to inspire:
_____
_____
_____

Thoughts to Sustain You – from Chris Ludwig

You read earlier that I've identified traits that are important to me, like - Courage, Grace, Trust, Flexibility, Humor, etc. and wrote those single words on post-its. I put them in places that I use every day — on top of the TV in our bedroom, near the phone, etc. So, when I go about my daily life and come across one of those virtues, I think about it. It's a great reminder to stay positive. I do the same when I come across an inspirational quote. Here are a few that are my favorites.

"Pleasure is always derived from somewhere outside you, while joy arises from within."-Eckhart Tolle

"Don't let life be about waiting for the storm to pass; make it about dancing in the rain."-Anonymous

"Faith is taking the first step, even when you don't see the whole staircase."-Martin Luther King

"Faith is being sure of what we hope for and certain of what we do not see."-Book of Hebrews

"Life isn't made up of every breath you take, but of moments that take your breath away."-Anonymous

Printed in Great Britain
by Amazon